# DATA QUEEN

Statistical Analysis Topics for Nursing Students

## First Edition

By Amy Moore

ISBN: 978-1-7331904-7-3
 Printed in the United States of America
First Printing, 2020

The copy editor was Qdmerit@fiverr.com.

The cover designer was Tinny Designs LLC, Design@TinnyGFX.com

# TABLE OF CONTENTS


## CHAPTER 1 DATA QUEEN FOR NURSING STUDENTS 1

IT IS YOUR PROJECT 1
MEDITATION TIME: ACCEPT THE CROWN 1
RESEARCH QUESTIONS AND YOUR STATS 3
PROPOSAL METHODOLOGY: THE BIG COMPROMISE 3
TYPICAL TEST STATISTICS IN NURSING PRACTICE 4
IMPORTANT FEATURES OF STATISTICAL REPORTING 5
LEARNING TO TALK STATISTICS 5
HOLDING COURT: PRESENT YOUR DATA 6
TALKING TO THE ROYAL COURT: FACULTY AND OTHER NURSING PROFESSIONALS 6

## CHAPTER 2 MEDITATION TIME—ACCEPT THE CROWN 7

THE SEVEN JEWELS OF THE CROWN 7
JEWEL #1: SAMPLE SIZE 7
JEWEL #2: SAMPLING METHOD 10
JEWEL #3: CHOOSING THE STATISTICAL METHOD 11
JEWEL #4: DATA COLLECTION 12
JEWEL #5: STATISTICAL SOFTWARE 13
JEWEL #6: STATISTICAL METHOD 14
JEWEL #7: RELATING TO THE STATISTICAL RESULTS 14
REFLECTIVE QUESTION 15

## CHAPTER 3 RESEARCH QUESTIONS AND YOUR STATS 16

WHAT WE WANT TO KNOW VS WHAT WE CAN OBTAIN IN 8-10 WEEKS 16
ANATOMY OF A RESEARCH QUESTION 17
RECHECK YOUR TARGET: WILL THE STATS ANSWER THE RESEARCH QUESTION? 18
PRACTICE PROBLEMS 19

**CHAPTER 4 PROPOSAL METHODOLOGY: THE BIG COMPROMISE 20**

SCENARIO #1: MY SITE WILL NOT LET ME CONDUCT MY STUDY 20
SCENARIO #2: SAMPLE SIZE NOT MET DUE TO CORONAVIRUS 21
SCENARIO #3: I DO NOT HAVE ACCESS TO PRE-PHASE DATA 21
SCENARIO #4: NO INCIDENCES TO RECORD FOR MY PROJECT 22
REFLECTIVE QUESTIONS 22

**CHAPTER 5 DATA STRUCTURE FOR TEST STATISTICS IN NURSING PRACTICE 23**

P-VALUE 23
PAIRED T-TEST 23
INDEPENDENT TWO SAMPLE T-TEST 25
ANOVA 25
CHI-SQUARE TEST 26
BINOMIAL TEST 27
PRACTICE PROBLEMS 27

**CHAPTER 6 APPROPRIATE USE OF GRAPHICS 29**

GRAPHS TO DISPLAY THE MEAN DIFFERENCE 29
GRAPHICS TO ILLUSTRATE PERCENTAGES 31
PRACTICE PROBLEMS 33

**CHAPTER 7 LEARN TO TALK STATISTICS 34**

LOOK IT UP FIRST 34
LEARN THE SYMBOLS 34
EXPLAIN IT TO SOMEONE ELSE 36
REFLECTIVE QUESTIONS 37

CHAPTER 8 HOLDING COURT: PRESENT YOUR DATA 38

YOU KNOW IT . . . BECAUSE YOU DID IT 38
HOW TO SAY, "I DON'T KNOW" WITHOUT SEEMING CLUELESS 38
STICK TO THE SLIDES 39
AN OFFENSE IS BETTER THAN NO DEFENSE 40
REFLECTIVE QUESTIONS 41

CHAPTER 9 TALKING TO THE ROYAL COURT: 42

FACULTY AND PEERS 42
HOW TO PREPARE FOR A DISCUSSION ABOUT YOUR DATA 42
FUTURE WORKS: PUBLICATIONS 43
REFLECTIVE QUESTIONS 44

APPENDICES 45

GLOSSARY 45

## Preface

*I wrote this book to help nursing students speak statistics. I hope this book empowers people to feel more confident about their involvement with data analytics. The book is designed to give practical advice regarding statistical topics. There are two types of exercises at the end of each chapter. Some problem sets are reflective and others are practical exercises. Please feel free to reach out to the author via email at amoore20@moorestat.com . You can also visit the author's shop at www.moorestat.com. After reading this book and working through the exercises, you should be familiar with the general expectations of the data flow process for statistical research. Beyond this book, I encourage you to add to your skill sets. Always remember you are a data queen!*

# CHAPTER 1

# DATA QUEEN FOR NURSING STUDENTS

## IT IS YOUR PROJECT

The other day I was speaking to a client who happened to be a Doctor of Nursing Practice (DNP) student. She was stressed about the task of performing her own quality improvement project. She went through a lengthy explanation as to why she is "not good at statistics." She repeated that negative mantra several times with a few expletives in between her words. I stayed silent on the other end of the phone, as this monologue was not for me. The student's admission was an exercise that I had grown accustomed to throughout my work. Often, people do not understand that their research project topic is more of a mystery than the statistical analysis. At some point, I responded to her with positive affirmations. I told her what I knew to be true. This is her project, and in the end, she will be the queen of her data. The data queen is someone who knows their project like the back of their hand. The *data queen* can explain the rationale of the study, the analysis, and the interpretation. The project sprouts from her creativity and knowledge of nursing. As we challenge ourselves through life experiences, we grow into who we were meant to be—the data queens.

## MEDITATION TIME: ACCEPT THE CROWN

It is time to get your head into the game. True, you do not know data, which would be problematic if this were solely a statistics graduate program. The subject involves a nursing degree, and the objective is to make an impact on health care within a nursing unit(s). All the statistics in the world cannot make an impact in the nursing field without your expertise. You bring a lot to the table. Nursing is your wheelhouse. Please accept the leadership position for the project. Accept the fact that you are the bridge between the data and nursing practice. So, it is time to take ownership and accountability for the data aspect of the project.

The mission is to make your data *sing* a narrative that answers the research question. If we were to outline the choreography of a quantitative DNP project, it would look something like Figure 1. The research question is clearly defined at the onset. The statistical tools must be defined for analysis. Sampling characteristics, sample size calculations, variable types, and statistical methodology should be part of the write-up of the project. The analysis will enable you to answer the research question.

FIGURE 1. TYPICAL DATA FLOW OF A DNP PROJECT

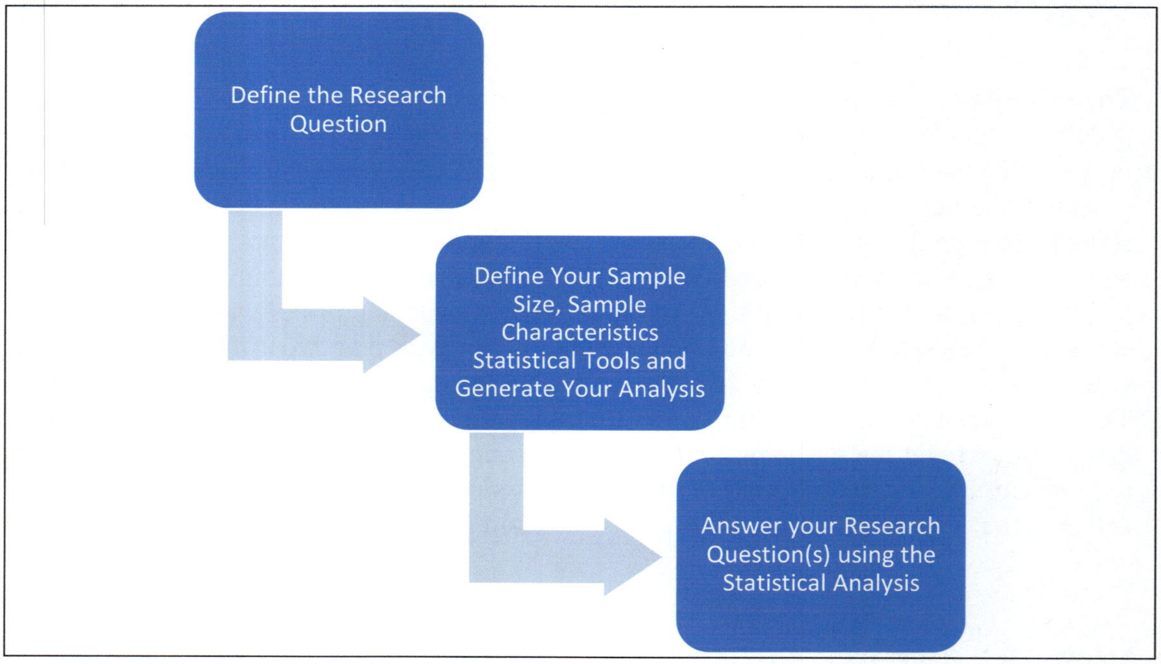


The data flow for statistical reports extends beyond nursing. It is a DNP requirement that you conduct research or a quality improvement performance project. But the undercurrent of data reporting is driven by statistical principles. Someone should be able to take your manuscript and duplicate the results using the same specifications. At some point in time, someone may want to implement your brilliant idea for their nursing units.

## RESEARCH QUESTIONS AND YOUR STATS

The data flow of a DNP project requires you to choose a research question that is answerable in an 8- to 10-week timeframe. If the project is focused on a rare event, it might take longer than two months to collect data. At the same time, it may not be feasible to collect voluminous data for a DNP project. Manual retrospective chart reviews require careful transcription of the data to a spreadsheet for further analysis. So, the research question should be measurable within an 8- to 10-week period. Sample size calculations can help estimate the size of your population, but you should also be aware of your facilities' limitation. If there are only 15 nursing participants for the project, that needs to be factored into your final calculations.

## PROPOSAL METHODOLOGY: THE BIG COMPROMISE

Sometimes we must factor in the working environment for the project. As previously expressed, there may be a shortage of project participants. You may discover that your nursing unit is so vigilant that there are no incidents to study for analysis. The proposal methodology is designed to help students navigate their project. In Table 1.1, the author has identified three scenarios which call for adjustments to your expectations of the project.

TABLE 1.1 POSSIBLE LIMITATIONS FOR A DNP PROJECT

| Scenario | Limitation | Possible Solution |
|---|---|---|
| The data collection does not coincide with the DNP proposal. A paired t-test must be performed for the project. | The spreadsheet has weekly data. | Conduct a paired t-test comparing the first and the last week of data. |
| The sample size estimation cannot be met. | There are only 10 nurses for a project that requires 40 participants. | Conduct a non-parametric test to compensate for the small sample size. |
| The outcome measure is immeasurable (missing or no data). | There are hardly any outcomes due to the nature of the dependent variable. | Descriptive statistics for any data with graphics. |

It is quite possible that one records more data than necessary. Pretest posttest analysis needs two measurements: (1) before and (2) after implementation. A paired t-test is just one example of a statistical method for analyzing mean differences between the two time periods. When you have too much data, it is still possible to provide graphics and description on any extraneous data.

### TYPICAL TEST STATISTICS IN DOCTOR NURSING PRACTICE

Most DNP projects study data pre and post intervention. Others report descriptive statistics for general reporting, especially if the intervention is novel. Every statistical analysis must include a summary of the dependent and independent variables under observation. Statistical summaries help one assess typical values that represent the sample and spread of the data. Interval variables are summarized using the mean and standard deviation. Categorical variables are represented with frequencies and percentages. Other statistical tests are listed in Table 1.2.

**TABLE 1.2 OTHER STATISTICAL TESTS FOR A DNP PROJECT**

| STATISTICAL METHODOLOGY | OBJECTIVE |
|---|---|
| Paired T-Test | To see if there is an overall improvement between pre and post intervention/implementation. |
| Independent Two Sample T-Test | To assess differences between two groups. |
| Chi-Square Test | To evaluate associations between two variables. |
| Mann-Whitney test | Non-parametric version of the independent samples t-test. |
| Wilcoxon Test | Non-parametric version of the paired t-test. |
| Binomial Test | To compare the rates between two time periods (example pre versus post). |
| ANOVA Test | Group comparison with more than two groups. |
| Cronbach's alpha | Used to test reliability of survey items in your survey tool. |

There are two types of statistical analysis: (1) descriptive and (2) inferential statistics. Descriptive statistics and frequencies are in every data report. Many quality improvement projects focus on the descriptive statistics for reporting. Inferential statistics help us draw conclusions about the sample data and population characteristics. Inferential analysis generates a likelihood or p-value. Probability tells us how likely we are to obtain the results in our statistical output. If your p-value is less than 0.05, the statistics associated with it are significant and worth reporting in detail. The overall premise of statistical reporting is to include only results which help you answer the research question (whether or not it is significant).

## IMPORTANT FEATURES OF STATISTICAL REPORTING

There are many ways data can be reported to demonstrate your knowledge of statistics. Your institution may provide the requirements for statistical reporting (narratives, tables, and figures). One should also be able to articulate the statistics in an oral presentation or informal conversation with faculty members. What it all comes down to is knowing what symbols and test statistics represent and convey in terms of your research question. Anyone can generate a paired t-test if the instructions are clearly outlined. However, one should also know how the statistics apply to the data in your DNP project. In other words, as the author of the manuscript, it is your job to bridge the gap between nursing and statistics.

## LEARNING TO TALK STATISTICS

You were not born speaking statistics in everyday language. It is a learned art form. If you were visiting a foreign country, you would prepare by learning a few smart phrases to survive your trip. The same is true with statistical analysis. The objective is to learn how to articulate your statistics in a manuscript, as well as in the DNP presentation. Table 1.3 shows a translation of basic concepts in statistics.

TABLE 1.3 TRANSLATION OF STATISTICS CONCEPTS

| Statistical Concept | English Translation |
|---|---|
| Confidence Interval | The range of values that may contain the true population parameter under study. |
| Alpha Criteria | Rejection criteria used to compare your generated p-value. |
| Mean | A typical value in your data. |
| Standard Deviation | The typical spread of your data around the mean. |
| R squared in Linear Regression | Percent of the variability explained by the statistical model. |
| Mean Difference | Difference between two means in a group comparison. |

## HOLDING COURT: PRESENT YOUR DATA

As you present your data to an audience, keep in mind that as the DNP researcher, you know more than anyone else. You know the variables collected as well as the limitations of the study. You can speak toward the statistical methodology and researched definitions associated with the results. Now it is show time. It is highly suggested that you know the details of the project like the back of your hand. There are ways to ensure that you are well prepared for a data presentation. There are exercises that one could perform with their peers to prepare for a presentation. We will explore a few options to help one feel confident with the DNP presentation.

## TALKING TO THE ROYAL COURT: FACULTY AND OTHER NURSING PROFESSIONALS

At some point you will need to discuss the project with faculty and other nursing professionals. In this conversation you need to come across as knowing every aspect of the project. You should be able to confidently discuss the details from the sample size to the statistical results. It is suggested that you have a detailed checklist of items to discuss with members of *the royal court.* Once you complete the proposal phase of the DNP project, there are specific characteristics that should be defined. The analysis phase of the DNP project has another set of characteristics that one should be able to articulate with faculty. Your ability to articulate various aspects of the project and answer questions will help facilitate your project.

# CHAPTER 2

## MEDITATION TIME—ACCEPT THE CROWN

Hey Queen! The mantra should be fully formed from this chapter. Every aspect of the DNP project should be fully understood by you. Because in the end, it is your research question(s) which will help make an impact on nursing. And it is genuinely believed that if you can anticipate what is needed for the statistics aspect of the project, you can reach some conclusions that are insightful, powerful, and influential for the field. Knowing what to expect is half the battle when it comes to claiming ownership of the statistics in your project. Breathe deeply for a time of reflection!

### THE SEVEN JEWELS OF THE CROWN

Several jewels of the crown should be familiar to the data queen. The first six gems are the following: sample size, sampling method, statistical method, data collection, statistical software, and statistical method. The final *ruby* is the ability to relate the statistical results to your nursing practice.

### JEWEL #1: SAMPLE SIZE

Sampling estimation is a slippery slope in nursing. Sometimes you cannot meet the adequate sample size for your project. Other times there is so much data that it is impossible to summarize it. Sample size is supposed to limit how much aggravation you must endure in the eight to ten weeks of the experience. Lot of nurses must juggle a heavy workload in addition to conducting the research or quality improvement project. Time is of the essence. So one must apply common sense with sample calculations. Sample size estimation is not needed for a descriptive study, such as a quality improvement project. However, sample size calculations are used when you are trying to infer something about the population under study. Inferencing requires a p-value statistic. It is that simple. And there are several types of sample size calculations. Each one has parameters which must be answered to get an accurate estimation. Table 2.1 shows examples of parameters across statistical methods.

**Table 2.1 Requirements of statistical methods**

| Statistical methods | Minimum Sample size parameters |
|---|---|
| Paired T-Test | Mean differences; standard deviation; effect size; alpha criteria; power |
| Independent Two Sample T-Test | Mean differences; effect size; alpha criteria; power |
| Fischer's Exact Test | Proportions; effect size; alpha criteria; Power |
| Pearson's Correlations | Effect size; alpha criteria; power; test statistic null hypothesis |

Sample size calculations should be based on the statistical method choice. Paired t-test requires a guestimate of the mean difference. If you believe the difference will be 5 units between the two time periods, then your mean difference is 5. Every sample size calculation will have an effect size, which is the influence on the outcome due to an intervention. The greater the differences between the groups, the larger effect size. In layman's terms, if you expect a sizeable improvement in the post intervention phase, the effect size will be large. Small effect sizes require a larger sample size to detect statistical significance. Effect size is determined by the researcher. The alpha criteria is another parameter which determines the significance level of the hypothesis test, typically set at 0.05. And the power of the test is the likelihood that your hypothesis testing is working correctly (for example: reject the null hypothesis when it is supposed to). The power of the test is usually set at 80% power.

There are free software packages that calculate effect size. G Power is a sample size calculator that can be downloaded to your computer. It is recommended that you verify the results with a professional. Sample size calculations are not trivial tasks. An over estimation may show faulty statistical significance. If there are not enough participants, the inference test may fail to detect findings. Figure 2.1 shows an example of a paired t-test calculation. As we fill out the fields in G Power, it is expected that we transfer our specifications to the proposal and final manuscript. That way someone of authority can take the numbers and verify the sample size.

FIGURE 2.1 EXAMPLE OF A PAIRED T-TEST CALCULATION IN G-POWER

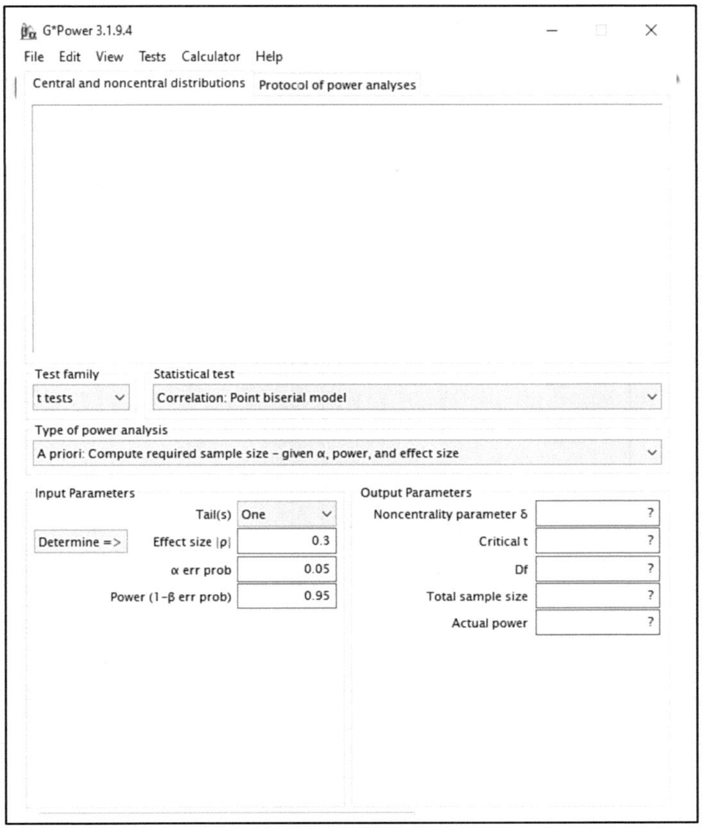


If you are conducting research, the sample size specification (effect size, power of the test, alpha, mean differences, etc.) should be included in the institutional review board (IRB) application, especially for cases where the project involves patient participants. It is also recommended that you disclose which statistical method is associated with the calculations. Vagueness will result in a blizzard of questions from your faculty. So, it is always helpful to be as transparent as possible. Attention to detail also helps to organize your thoughts concerning the project itself.

Now if it is a quality improvement project, you need to define how many medical staff are participants. In any case, the sample size should be defined within reason. If your unit of measure is nurses and there are only ten medical staff, that is the sample size limitation.

## JEWEL #2: SAMPLING METHOD

A sampling method is a technique for gathering data. The sampling approach will determine how you treat the data. A convenience sampling method describes the process of collecting accessible data for a period. Local patients or medical staff are solicited to participate in the project. It is also referred to as a non-probabilistic sampling, where probability is not factored into the method of selection. Patient participants from a clinic would be an example of convenient sampling. Probability sampling ensures that each member of the population has an equal chance of being selected for the study. Project participants could be randomly selected using Statistical Package for the Social Scienes (SPSS), for instance, to avoid bias. In layman's terms, we do not want to skew our results by subjectively selecting cases that will yield a particular outcome. In Figure 2.1, we see the random sampling generator in SPSS (found under the *select cases* option). The software gives you the option of randomly selecting a percentage of the cases or an exact number of participants. However, most DNP projects are focused on populations that are easily accessible, or convenient samples.

FIGURE 2.1 RANDOM SELECTION SAMPLING FOR SPSS

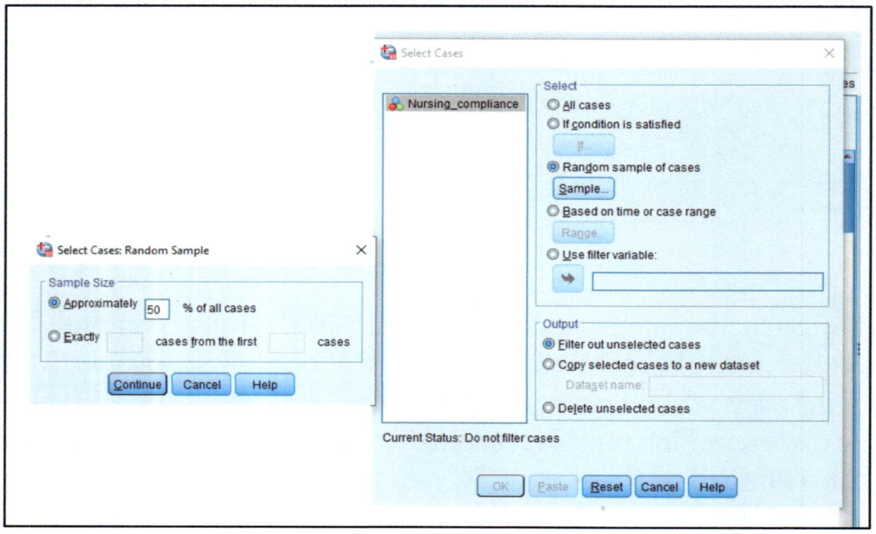


It is important to define the sampling method because it dictates the statistical methods used in the project. Convenient sampling methods should be paired with non-parametric statistics where you can analyze the data without factoring in the normal distribution of the sample. Probabilistic sampling is associated with parametric statistics, such as, student t-tests or linear regression. In layman's terms, you should not use a convenient sample to generalize the population with a parametric test. If you perform a parametric test on a nursing unit, for example, you cannot assume the results can infer anything beyond the sample. The fundamental difference between parametric and non-parametric statistics is the probability distribution. Non-parametric testing will not analyze the actual data; it focuses on the order of the values. Non-parametric statistics focus on the magnitude and direction of the data. Parametric statistics link the values to a likelihood to conduct predictions. Table 2.2 lists a few parametric and non-parametric statistical tests.

TABLE 2.2 PARAMETRIC AND NON-PARAMETRIC TESTS

| Parametric Tests | Non-Parametric Equivalent |
|---|---|
| Pearson's Correlation | Spearman Correlation |
| Independent Two Sample t | Mann-Whitney U |
| One-Way Repeated Measures ANOVA | Freidman Test |
| Logistic Regression | Chi-Square Test |

NOTE

The author makes a loose comparison between the idea of an *association* versus a *relationship*. The statistics for assessing a relationship involve the full picture with all the variables that influence the outcome. The association is a more general analysis that focuses on the two factors under study. A Chi-Square test will tell you there is an association. A logistic regression will provide the odds of an outcome occurring given several independent variables.

## JEWEL #3: CHOOSING THE STATISTICAL METHOD

The statistical method is the way in which the data will be analyzed to answer the questions raised in the project. The dependent variable type gives you the first hint as to which test statistic is the most appropriate. Table 2.2 shows variable types and their associated family of test statistics.

TABLE 2.2 VARIABLE TYPES AND FAMILY OF STATISTICS

| Dependent Variable Type | Family of Test Statistics |
|---|---|
| Nominal or Ordinal | Chi Square; Binomial Test; Fisher's Exact Test; Factorial Analysis |
| Interval | Student t-tests; Independent t-tests; Paired t-tests Linear Regression, ANOVA, MANOVA |

If there is difficulty with determining the dependent variable type, sketch it. How many possible answer choices are you expecting in the data? If the variable has only two answer choices, that is nominal data, specifically a binomial value. Variables that have measurements for data, such as blood pressure or decimal measurements, are interval variables. When you visualize the data for collection, it ensures that the statistical methodology matches the intent. The manuscript should reflect careful planning and critical thinking. Ordinal data would not be used for a Pearson's correlation statistic. Interval data would not be analyzed for a chi square test. Everything must make sense to execute the project successfully. The DNP proposal is the playbook for every aspect of the work. Use it wisely.

### JEWEL #4: DATA COLLECTION

It was previously suggested that you plan the data format at the proposal stage of the project. The variables in the spreadsheet should represent either the outcome measure or an independent variable. What happens if you skip the planning of data collection? Planning at each step keeps your mind clear and focused on the task. If the data is collected without a strategy, variables may not be compatible with the test statistic of choice; the project may leave out important information, and you may not complete the project successfully.

In terms of data collection tools, most people prefer Excel spreadsheets. It really depends on the data source. If the data is coming from retrospective chart reviews, Excel is a practical choice. Excel is software that comes with Microsoft Office. The column headers serve as variable names and the rows represent subject participants. Table 2.3 shows an example of data in Excel.

TABLE 2.3 DATA IN EXCEL

| | A | B | C |
|---|---|---|---|
| 1 | Nurse ID | pre score | post score |
| 2 | 1 | 9 | 10 |
| 3 | 2 | 5 | 8 |
| 4 | 3 | 4 | 11 |
| 5 | 4 | 11 | 12 |
| 6 | | | |

The column headers should be in the first row of the Excel file. Other statistical software packages require short column headers; it is suggested that it be a length of 7 characters at maximum. The reason is that people tend to use multiple statistical software languages to analyze their data. It is common practice to pull the data from Excel to SPSS. Aside from the column headers or variable names, one should choose a familiar statistical software. Why? Because the author strongly recommends that the DNP researcher be able to duplicate the statistics results on their own. Why? At some point, you may have to defend your analysis choice.

## JEWEL #5: STATISTICAL SOFTWARE

Statistical software receptacles for data entry should not be confused with more robust packages such as SPSS. Survey monkey can summarize the data without much effort. More complex statistics can be done in SPSS, Statistical Analysis Software (SAS), Statistics and Data Software (STATA), STATCrunch, or R software to name a few. Again, you should use the platform in your wheelhouse instead of reinventing the wheel. SPSS is like Excel and it has a user-friendly interface. Some DNP programs may require that you learn a computer language, such as, R or SAS. If you want to learn more about those languages, please check out *Getting Your Feet Wet with R*, *The R Funk: A Beginner's Guide to Creating R Functions*, and *Out of the Box Statistics Workbook Using SAS*.

### JEWEL #6: STATISTICAL METHOD

Sometimes we choose a statistical method that does not turn out well. Maybe our sample size is too small. Or the variable format must be converted to another variable type for a different analysis. Flexibility is sometimes a necessity. If you collect data that looks unfavorable, the faculty may decide to change the outcome variable format. If it is advisable to measure something as categorical rather than interval, a change in the statistical approach may be required. The key is not to freak out. Keep your composer and navigate towards a different goal.

### JEWEL #7: RELATING TO THE STATISTICAL RESULTS

The most under-rated step of analysis is the translation from numbers to nursing practice. Statistical interpretation is the process of making numbers digestible for non-technical people. Your role is to answer the research questions raised in the discussion section of the manuscript. Table 2.3 shows examples of statistics that do not answer the research question.

**TABLE 2.3 RESEARCH QUESTIONS AND ANSWER STATUS**

| Research Question | Test Statistics Used | Question Answered Yes or No? |
|---|---|---|
| Is there an increase in smoking cessation among patients with lung cancer? | Mean and Standard Deviation | No. Smoking cessation is an event which must be recorded as binominal (yes or no). |
| Is there an association between smoking status and the type of cessation program (1, 2 or 3)? | Binomial Test | No. Associations are answered with the chi square test. |
| Is there a relationship between the outcome measurement, smoking status, and age of patient? | Linear Regression | Yes |
| Is there a difference in weight loss on program A versus Program B for obese patients? | Independent Two Sample t Test | Yes |

Knowing the variable type and corresponding statistics will ensure that research questions are answered appropriately. Unless it is a score, smoking cessation is analyzed with the mean and standard deviation. If you have degrees of cessation (reduction in packs a day) then it could be an interval variable type. Any time a research topic measures degrees of association, it is performed with a proportion test, such as the chi square statistic. Binomial tests are focused on the difference in the rates instead of the variables. Relationships between multiple independent and dependent variables can be assessed with linear regression if the outcome measure is interval.

Many times, we start our travels in a clueless haze, because the experience is new to us. The descriptions of the jewels of the crown is meant to shine light on what is needed to complete a manuscript or data report. Awareness of the *crown* will facilitate your journey through the process. Hopefully, the following chapters will provide insight related to the rocks and boulders that may impede the path.

## REFLECTIVE QUESTIONS

1. How many crown jewels do you possess?
2. Do you know the format of the variables that will help to answer the research question?
3. What statistical software is in your wheelhouse?
4. Have you planned data collection for the project?
5. Is your sampling method random or is it the convenient sampling method?
6. Is your project a quality improvement project or a research study?

# CHAPTER 3

# RESEARCH QUESTIONS AND YOUR STATS

In this book the term *research question* refers to the objectives of the project or manuscript. The purpose of the research question is to assess a demographic, over a period, with outcomes and prognostic factors. If the topic is quantitative in nature, it includes dependent and independent variables. The variables will be used to collect data in a format. As evidence is gathered through data entry or query, we gain insight on the research question. As we identify a statistical method, certain words or phrases will trigger the need for an analytical procedure. The data is not always going support the objectives of the topic. Not every scenario yields statistical significance. There may be limitations to your study environment that negatively influence the results. The key is to have an open mind when it comes to answering the research questions with your work.

## WHAT WE WANT TO KNOW VS WHAT WE CAN OBTAIN IN 8-10 WEEKS

Some research questions take longer to answer than others due to the nature of the data. If the project is on a time constraint, it is wise to choose a topic that is answerable in 8 to 10 weeks. Suppose you choose incidence of baby falls in a nursing unit. Historically, your unit has had more than 2 falls in a quarter. If you know it will take more than 10 weeks to obtain data, then maybe baby falls is not a good research topic. Table 3.1 shows research topics and their limitations in terms of data. If the study period is longer than 90 days, that means it will be necessary to wait for the data to be collected in that timeframe. Other scenarios call for re-defining the research question to focus on more specific details. You cannot include every emergency room scenario. It helps to focus on a unit of measurement, patients or medical staff, and an outcome of interest. How long will it take to collect the data? Will you collect it manually or through a computerized query? If there are a few hundred cases, a manual review is a feasible approach. But if there are thousands of subjects, it might be too much for one person.

**TABLE 3.1 PROBLEMATIC RESEARCH QUESTION**

| RESEARCH QUESTIONS | ISSUE |
|---|---|
| Is there is a decrease in the frequency of 90 day re-admissions for stroke victims? | The time limit for the project is two months. |
| Does the *M* screening tool reduce the frequency of emergency visits? | Too general a topic. It needs to be narrowed down to a specific type of emergency visit, demographic, and outcome. |
| Does the training program reduce contaminated blood samples in hospital X? | Sample size could potentially be too large and cumbersome for a 10-week study. |

There is a way to execute projects with challenging data scenarios. If the pre-phase data collect cannot be obtained in person, one could use retrospective chart reviews. It is advisable to investigate if there is data available in electronic format. A simple data query (de-identified) could be a solution to the problem. Telehealth projects are a viable option at the facility. Some place may even provide data to analyze for the purposes of simulating a project.

## ANATOMY OF A RESEARCH QUESTION

A research question should include a unit of measurement: patient or medical staff. If you are studying nursing compliance, then nursing staff should be the focus of the research question. If there is an intervention, it should mention the objectives of the topic. The most difficult concept to grasp is the outcome measure. The outcome measure is the event under study. It is the dependent variable in all your statistical models. And it will help to determine if the project was successful. The time factor is 8 to 10 weeks for a DNP project. In this book, we will not explore the time it takes to obtain a particular outcome as an analysis parameter.

**RECHECK YOUR TARGET: WILL THE STATS ANSWER THE RESEARCH QUESTION?**

As the project progresses, it is helpful to ensure that the results will answer the research question. If the assessment involves an improvement between two periods, the statistics should have two outcome measurements (pre and post phases). If you are comparing two groups (men and women, for example), there should be two sets of calculations that represent the subgroups. If the inclusion criteria focuses on diabetic patients, there should be no non-diabetics in the sample population. We will look at statistical methodology in Chapter 5. Table 3.2 shows examples where the statistical results do not answer the research question. The table also shows a better question that is compatible with the original statistical method.

TABLE 3.2

| Statistical Method | Research Question | Issue | Better Research Question |
|---|---|---|---|
| Paired T-test | Is there a relationship between the patients survey score and the nurse's compliance rate? | The statistical method, a paired t-test, calls for two outcome measures for one unit of measure (all nurses or all patients). | Is there a difference in the patient's survey score after the implementation of the X tool? |
| ANOVA (Analysis of Variance) | Does the gender of a patient affect the compliance rate? | Gender could be two possible outcomes (female versus male). The ANOVA procedure is for more than two groups. | Does patient's race affect the compliance rate? |
| Chi-Square Test | Does smoking cessation decrease blood pressure in adult patients? | Blood pressure is an interval measure. If you are assessing the difference, it should not be a statistic for count data. | Is there an association between smoking status and the blood pressure status (high or low)? |

The research question should match the statistical method which is in the manuscript proposal. There are test statistics for interval outcome measurements such as the Paired t-test and the ANOVA (Analysis of Variance). Key phrases such as *the difference* will suggest that you are dealing with an interval variable. The chi square test, an association statistic, is for cases where the data is a frequency and percent. In the next chapter, we will explore the statistical expectations of a quantitative project.

**PRACTICE PROBLEMS**

1. Identify possible variables that could be obtained to answer the research topic.
   a. Weight loss for obese diabetic patients.
   b. Improvements in nursing knowledge score for the chlamydia diagnostic tool.
   c. Implementation of the nutrition X program to promote healthier food choices in breast cancer patients?

2. Identify the variable format of the answers from #1.

3. Identify the statistical methodology that should be performed based on your response to #2.

4. What type of statistic will be used to answer your response to number #3? Here are your choices:

   a. A mean and standard deviation.
   b. More than one set of means and standard deviations.
   c. A P-value.
   d. Frequency and percentages with bar charts.
   e. Some other method. Specify________________________________.

5. What is the variable format of the dependent variable for each statistical method?
   a. ANOVA
   b. Mann-Whitney U test
   c. Kruskal-Wallis
   d. Paired t-test
   e. Linear regression
   f. Logistic regression
   g. Chi-Square test

# CHAPTER 4

# PROPOSAL METHODOLOGY: THE BIG COMPROMISE

The proposal phase of your manuscript is the most important milestone of the entire project. The planning stage of the project defines the research question(s), statistical method, sample size calculation, unit of measure for data collection, the outcome measures, and any other supporting parameters. As the author works with clients, it is evident that students face re-curing struggles. There are situations where we carefully plan our proposal methodology, and yet life throws us a curve ball. As things occur during the project, one must adjust and come up with feasible solutions that do not impede progress. Here are a few scenarios and possible solutions.

## SCENARIO #1: MY SITE WILL NOT LET ME CONDUCT THE PROJECT

It is upsetting when a hospital decides to delay the progress on a student's project. As a former statistician and an IRB reviewer in a hospital setting, the author understands why projects are delayed by scientific committees. There are several reasons for it. Sometimes the resistance has to do with personnel at the site who do not understand the DNP process. You may come across a situation where there is a personality clash. Sometimes personality conflicts can be mitigated with the intervention of decision makers. Other times, it may be that your project lacks specific detail. Hospitals can be strict about who is qualified to conduct their work on-site. Other reasons for a slow approval decision can be related to factors that have nothing to do with the project's proposal. Maybe it is expected that you only use hospital's resources. One should do critical thinking about the issue. You work in a hospital where all data reporting must be monitored within that site. Your work will be published for the literary community. The site may have structures in place that ensure the data is adequately reported in the project. So, push back should be expected from the site. You are triggering some form of hospital protocol by the scientific committee which meets on a schedule. In other situations, students experienced delays in their proposal acceptance, after hiring an independent contractor. Outside contractors are scrutinized by sites that have personnel who perform similar job functions. One must accept three things: (1) your educational journey is important, and (2) the data must be worth the fight, (3) where the project is conducted is your choice. There may be other sites which are more amenable to your ideas. The downside to sticking it out may result in an incomplete project or delays in graduation. Or you may choose to abide by the preferences of that hospital. At the end of the day, the choice rests in your hands.

### SCENARIO #2: SAMPLE SIZE NOT MET DUE TO CORONAVIRUS

As we become a virtual environment with the pandemic, a lot of nursing projects have been disrupted due to the coronavirus. Non-parametric statistics are useful for cases where the sample size calculation falls short of expectations. If you obtained 15 instead of 35 patients for a paired t-test, it might be possible to use a Wilcoxon test, a non-parametric version of the paired t-test. Non-parametric statistics make it possible to analyze irregular sample sizes. If the project is focused on process quality improvement, then the sample size is not as important. One could conduct a descriptive analysis with graphical displays and interpret any visual trends in the data. If you have not yet collected data, it might be feasible to pivot the topic. Some professors have provided secondary data for analysis. Other institutions have recommended case series which require a smaller sample size. Maybe there is a topic that does not require in-person data collection. Again, it depends on how passionate you are about the topic.

### SCENARIO #3: I DO NOT HAVE ACCESS TO PRE-PHASE DATA

It may be hard to obtain data before the implementation phase, especially when the intervention is new and innovative. If no one has used the tool before, it may seem impossible to perform a comparison of pre to post data. New implementation tools do not have pre-phase data. It is the author's preference to avoid situations where a pre-post comparison is implemented and only the post data is available for collection. However, there have been studies which compensate for the missing information. One may decide to run a descriptive study to assess how the data behaves with the new intervention. Observational projects can be very insightful for future publications. Or it is possible to choose statistics which do not require individual information about the pre-phase period. If you have access to a database, it is possible to query for aggregate data. Rates can be generated to determine if there was an overall change between the two phases, but if the goal is to compare individual cases between pre and post data, both periods must be present.

### SCENARIO #4: NO INCIDENCES TO RECORD FOR MY PROJECT

Some data is hard to obtain because there are no cases to evaluate due to several factors. If the outcome measure is a rare event, it may influence the sample size. Typically, rare events are seen in quality improvement projects where the focus is on the performance of medical staff.

The rate of data collection should be monitored on a regular basis. If a week goes by and no data is collected in the spreadsheet, it does not mean no data exists for the project. There may be a reason why the data was not recorded for that instance. It is suggested that one does not wait until the end of the project to inspect missing information. Once the study period has ended, it may be difficult to fix problematic cases.

### REFLECTIVE QUESTIONS

1. What is the reason you are experiencing delays with the project? Is the issue with the school or the site?
2. Is the data obtainable through an electronic query?
3. Are you using a validated implementation tool with available pre-data?
4. If the sample size is impossible to collect, can you pick a new topic with better data?
5. Is your objective to graduate, make an impact on the field of nursing, or both?
6. Are you well-informed on the available resources on the site?
7. If you answered *yes* to #6, do you feel adequately supported by the personnel at the site?

# CHAPTER 5

# DATA STRUCTURE FOR TEST STATISTICS IN NURSING PRACTICE

There are statistical tests for use on DNP projects. It can be challenging to decide which test to use for a scenario. It depends on several factors. If you are conducting a descriptive analysis, there is no p-value associated with the results. Descriptive analysis is a statistical summary for interval variables. Frequency and percentages are performed for categorical variables (nominal or ordinal) in the data; however, if one is trying to infer something about the population, then a p-value should be reported in the analysis. Some statistical methodologies will give you a probability that your results are statistically significant. Once you recognize which test statistic is appropriate, then the spreadsheet should be mapped out with the dependent and independent variables. The data structure is specific to the test statistic.

## P-VALUE

The p-value is a statistic that indicates the likelihood that your data is meaningless and at random. In other words, a low p-value suggests it is less likely that you just happened to find data with those values. A high p-value may suggest that another attempt at the project would yield different results. Data can be interpreted as *garbage* if the p-value is higher than 5% or 0.05. Your alpha criteria set the threshold for rejecting the notion that the intervention made an impact. The alpha is the acceptable level for detecting statistical significance. Some publications will describe the alpha criteria lower than 1% depending upon the results.

## PAIRED T-TEST

The paired t-test is a test statistic used to assess the mean difference between two periods. It is not uncommon to compare the data before and after implementation of an intervention. The outcome measure is an interval format (scaled measurement). The objective is to show that the intervention had an influence on the post implementation data. If your data is not statistically significant, then there is no difference between the periods. Table 5.1 shows the SPSS output for a paired t-test. The data structure of a paired t-test must contain two dependent variables (pre versus post) and the subject id (med staff or patient). Table 5.1 shows the data structure for a paired t-test.

TABLE 5.1 PAIRED T-TEST DATA

| ID | Pre Score | Post Score |
|---|---|---|
| 1 | 20 | 15 |
| 2 | 5 | 10 |
| 3 | 10 | 2 |
| 4 | 22 | 4 |
| 5 | 4 | 13 |
| 6 | 25 | 23 |
| 7 | 15 | 25 |

The pre and post scores serve as the dependent variables. If you collected interim data (between the two periods) it is suggested that you make a graph of weekly measurements. Figure 5.1 shows weekly data in a bar chart.

Figure 5.1

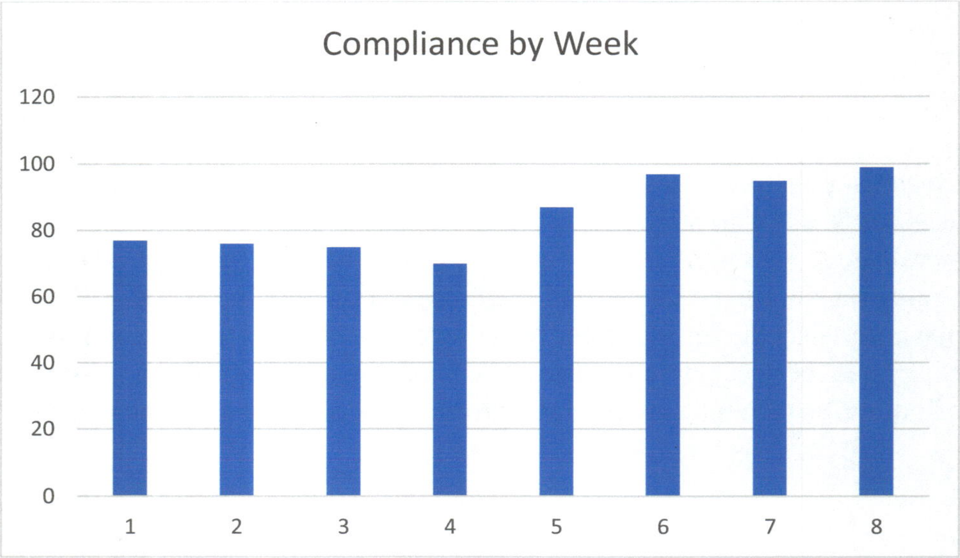


The first and last week of the project can be used for this analysis. Week one could serve as the pre-phase period versus week 8 (post implementation phase).

### INDEPENDENT TWO SAMPLE T-TEST

Another comparison analysis is the independent two-sample t-test which looks for differences in the means between two groups. More importantly, you are trying to suggest that the sub-groups are coming from two entirely different populations. The test statistic assumes no participants are present in both the pre- and post-implementation phase. A participant can only be represented in one group. The objective is to show that the intervention influenced the participants during the post-implementation phase. Table 5.2 is an example of the data for an independent two-sample t-test.

TABLE 5.2 INDEPENDENT TWO-SAMPLE T-TEST

| ID | Patient_Scores | Phase |
|---|---|---|
| 1 | 22 | Pre |
| 2 | 33 | Pre |
| 3 | 24 | Post |
| 4 | 56 | Post |

The dependent variable of an independent two-sample t-test should represent one column of the data. Table 5.2 shows the dependent variable as patient scores with the phase indicating the sub-group. The phase will indicate whether the participant belonged to the pre- or post-implementation phase. There should be one id for each individual and no duplicate information. In other words, one should not be presented in both groups.

### ANOVA

The analysis of variance (ANOVA) is the analysis of an outcome measurement when the independent variable has more than two categories. It is an extension of the independent sample t-test. Participants are classified in one of the comparison groups. Table 5.3 shows an example of the data for an ANOVA test statistic.

TABLE 5.3 EXAMPLE OF AN ANOVA DATA STRUCTURE

| ID | Patient_Scores | Race |
|---|---|---|
| 1 | 3.4 | Asian |
| 2 | 3.2 | African America |
| 3 | 3.0 | Other |
| 4 | 2.3 | Caucasian |
| 5 | 2.1 | Asian |

It is important to note that the sample size estimation should be calculated for each scenario. The examples only demonstrate the structure of the data. ANOVA's cannot generate statistics if there is only one person in each category. You will see this issue with SPSS or any statistical software.

### CHI-SQUARE TEST

The chi square test is used to assess associations between categorical variables, both the outcome measurement and the independent variables. The analysis is focused on the counts and percentages in each cell. Data preparation for a chi square test assumes that you have nominal or ordinal values. Table 5.4 shows the data structure for patients diagnosed with a stress disorder (yes or no) and by gender (male or female). Bother variables are nominal format.

TABLE 5.4 AN EXAMPLE OF DATA STRUCTURE FOR A CHI SQUARE TEST

| ID | GENDER | STRESS DISORDER |
|---|---|---|
| 1 | MALE | YES |
| 2 | FEMALE | NO |
| 3 | FEMALE | YES |
| 4 | MALE | NO |
| 5 | MALE | YES |
| 6 | FEMALE | YES |
| 7 | MALE | NO |

## BINOMIAL TEST

The binomial test is used to compare rates pre and post implementation. The test statistic was mentioned to demonstrate its usefulness during the COVID Pandemic. If the pre data rate is known, it can be used as the null hypothesis for your binomial test. The post data should be in binomial format, with just two possible answer choices (preferably 0 or 1 values). Table 5.5 shows the data structure that is needed for a binomial test.

TABLE 5.5 DATA STRUCTURE FOR A BINOMIAL TEST

| ID | Outcome |
|---|---|
| 1 | Yes |
| 2 | No |
| 3 | Yes |
| 4 | No |
| 5 | Yes |
| 6 | Yes |
| 7 | No |

The binomial test statistic will tell you if the rates are statistically different from each other. The test counts the number of *Yes* answer choices in the post-implementation phase, but you can apply this statistic to other periods (week 8 versus week 10 data). It is also good for cases where you have aggregate data, where there are no individual-level entries available.

## PRACTICE PROBLEMS

1. Identify the statistical method that could be performed based on the data structure of the file.

a.

| ID | Dehydration Status of Patient |
|---|---|
| 1 | Yes |
| 2 | No |
| 3 | Yes |
| 4 | No |
| 5 | Yes |
| 6 | Yes |
| 7 | No |

b.

| ID | Personnel | Implementation of Tool |
|---|---|---|
| 1 | Nurse | Yes |
| 2 | Provider | No |
| 3 | Provider | Yes |
| 4 | Nurse | No |
| 5 | Provider | Yes |
| 6 | Provider | Yes |
| 7 | Nurse | No |

c.

| ID | Personnel | Implementation of Tool | Age |
|---|---|---|---|
| 1 | Nurse | Yes | 20 |
| 2 | Provider | No | 40 |
| 3 | Provider | Yes | 42 |
| 4 | Nurse | No | 23 |
| 5 | Provider | Yes | 27 |
| 6 | Provider | Yes | 35 |
| 7 | Nurse | No | 45 |

# CHAPTER 6

# APPROPRIATE USE OF GRAPHICS

Graphics are a requirement for data reporting in most institutions. It demonstrates the highlights of the analysis performed in the summary or inferential statistics. Illustrations are based on variable type (categorical or scaled measurement). Some graphical displays are more appropriate than others in terms of illustrating differences in group comparisons. Sometimes a statistician will choose a graph because of personal preference. Bar charts are especially useful for showing mean differences between groups. Linear relationships between variables are studied with scatterplot data. Graphics are supposed to accent your data tables and narrative. Too many graphs may be confusing for the reader. The focus should be to provide graphics that help you answer the research questions raised in the publication.

## GRAPHS TO DISPLAY THE MEAN DIFFERENCE

The mean difference is a statistic that is calculated when you have interval data, measurements that are based on a continuous scale from zero to infinity. Weight and blood pressure are examples of interval variables. The mean statistic gives you an idea of how the values are *behaving* on average. In a graph, you want to convey the magnitude of the difference between pre and post. The bar chart is an excellent graph to display mean differences. Figure 6.1 shows the mean difference between two periods. In the figure, the pre phase has a higher mean. The mean difference is in favor of the pre phase due to the trends in the graph. Once the data pattern is recognized, it is up to the DNP researcher to relate it to the objectives of the project. Did you achieve success with the implementation of the intervention? Looking at Figure 6.1, if you had hoped to achieve lower results in the post period, the answer is *yes*. If we were expecting higher results in the post period, then we can conclude that our project was not successful. The expectations of the project determine how the graphs are interpreted for the viewing audience.

FIGURE 6.1 MEAN DIFFERENCES WITH BAR CHARTS

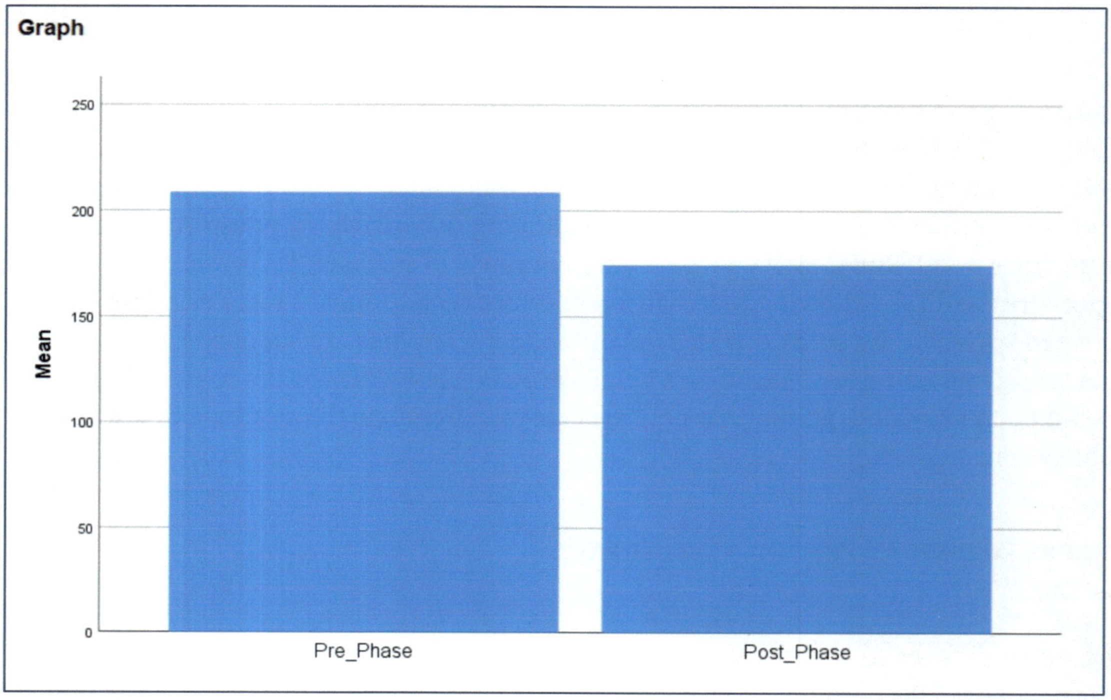


It is valuable to note that the standard deviation should be reported in the narrative or table of choice, but it is not always included in graphs to illustrate mean difference. The author tends not to make standard deviation the focal point for a mean difference statistical analysis, but it is appropriate to report the spread of the data, the standard deviation, for narratives.

It is possible to illustrate the confidence intervals of the data around the means. Error bars can be used for assessing the data spread for each period. Confidence intervals also suggest statistical significance of the data. If the confidence intervals do not overlap, then there is a statistically significant difference between the two groups. Figure 6.2 is an example of a graph with errors bars, which is appropriate for an independent sample t-test. We see that the two groups do not share any values in common, and we can assume the p-value is statistically significant.

FIGURE 6.2 GROUP COMPARISON WITH CONFIDENCE INTERVALS

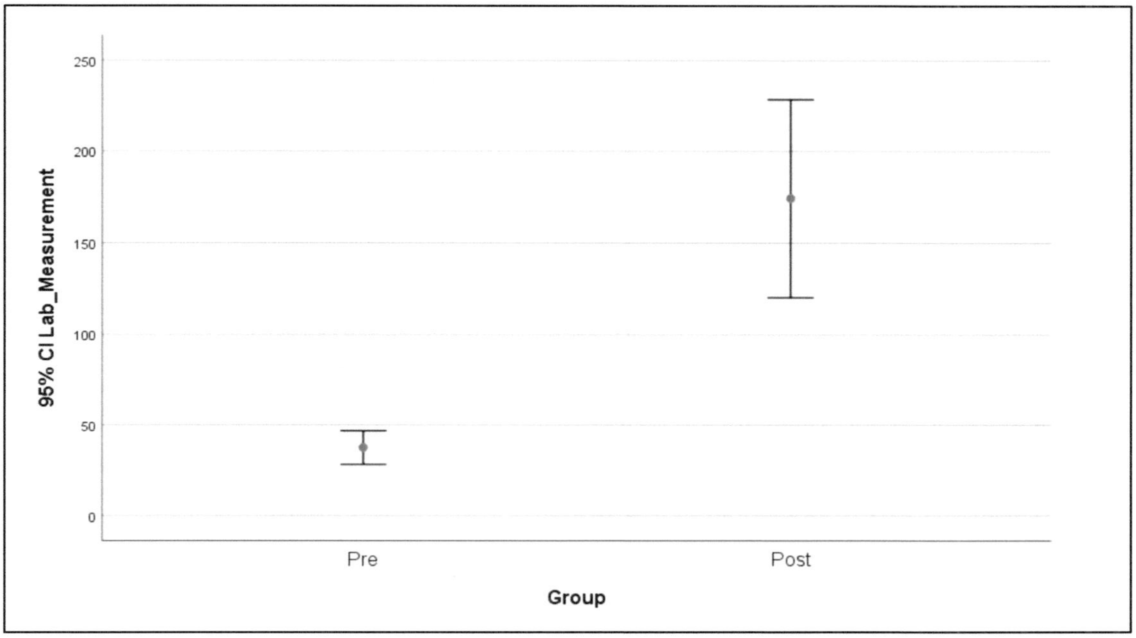


**GRAPHICS TO ILLUSTRATE PERCENTAGES**

There are graphs specifically for frequencies and percentages. Bar charts are used to illustrate categorical data where each level represents a characteristic. Figure 6.3 shows a bar chart for gender, nominal variables. As long as the percentage is greater than zero, the data will be visible in the graph. It is not possible to illustrate a quantity equal to zero. If your pre period has no data, a table of the percentages can be used to capture 0%. Another approach for count data is to use a pie chart. It is possible to annotate the chart and add percentages for the sub-groups within the graph. The key is to choose an illustration that is readable for the viewer. If there are too many categories, interpretation could be difficult.

FIGURE 6.3 BAR CHART OF THE CATEGORICAL VARIABLE GENDER

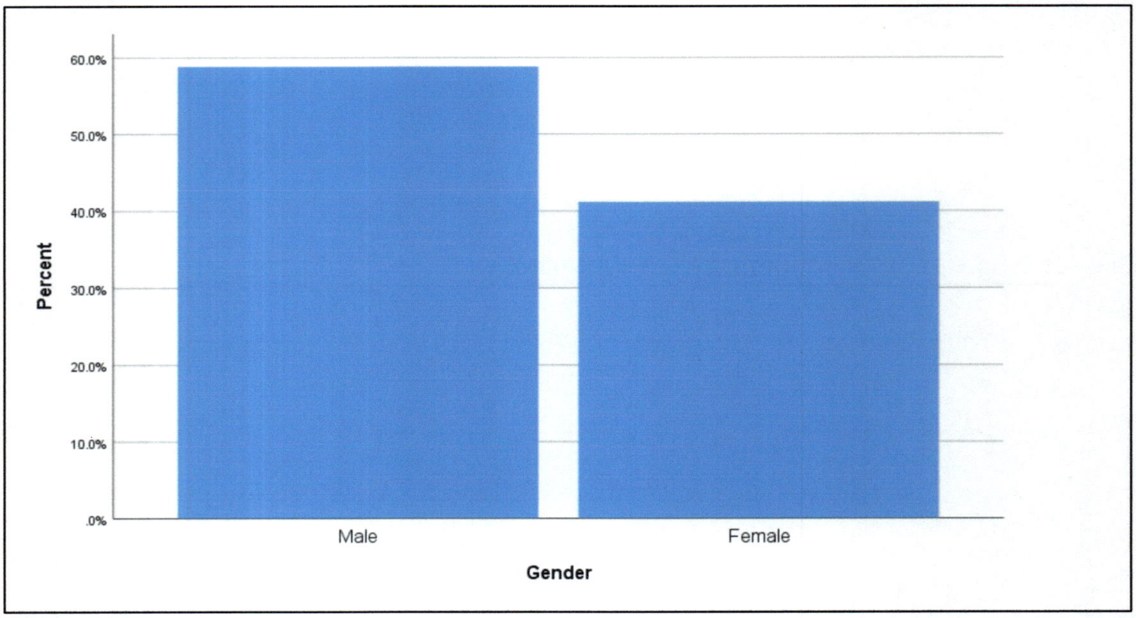


FIGURE 6.4 PIE CHART OF THE CATEGORICAL VARIABLE, GENDER

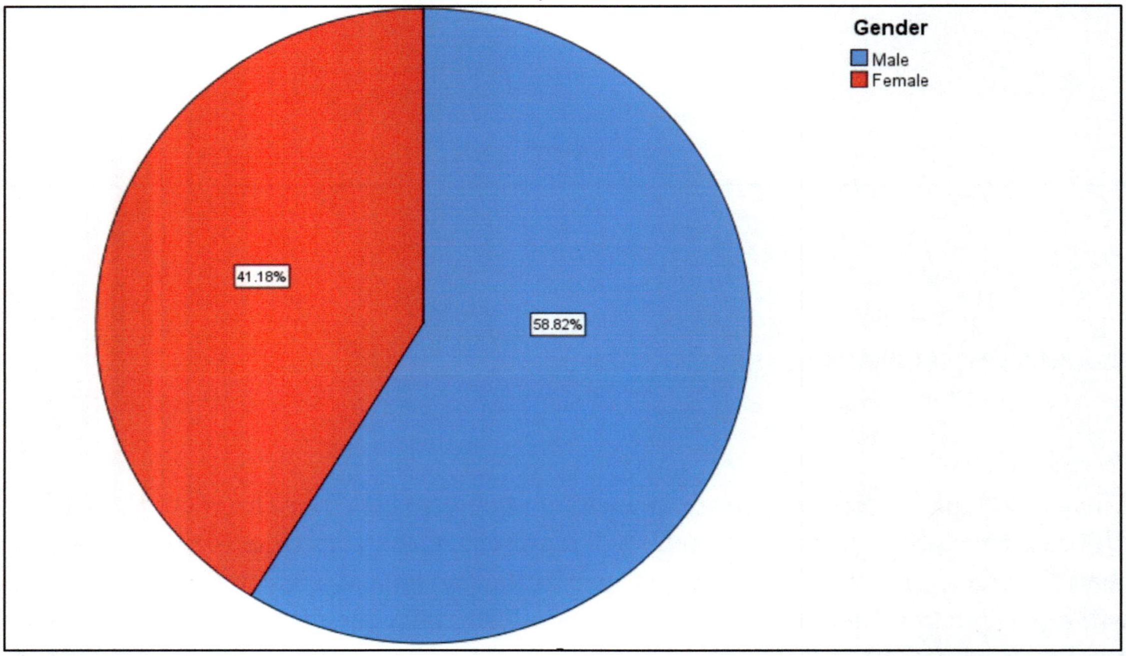

## Practice Problems

1. Identify the type of variable used to illustrate the graph.

    a. Patients' fall score (pre versus post)
    b. Number of tracheotomies (pre versus post)
    c. Number of contaminated blood samples
    d. Mean cholesterol (pre versus post)
    e. SBAR score (pre versus post)
    f. Frequency of readmitted stroke patients

2. Name the type of graphs needed for your answer to #1.
3. What graph could be used to illustrate weekly nursing compliance of an implementation tool?
4. Reflective question: should a graph that does not support the research topic be included in the publication?

# CHAPTER 7

# LEARN TO TALK STATISTICS

If you needed to speak French for a presentation, you would study the French language. You must learn the language of statistics to communicate effectively with others who speak it. Conversations about statistics seem more natural if you know the vocabulary. If you cannot articulate the data, then people will scrutinize the results. The more questions that arise from the project, the harder it will be to achieve final project approval. It also helps to remember that you are not an imposter pretending to do research that was never performed. You did the work. So let's become more familiar with the language of statistics.

## LOOK IT UP FIRST

If there is a symbol or statistical output that makes no sense, one should research it on the internet. It is customary to look up phrases that are hard to pronounce and seem to have no meaning. Do you need to learn everything there is to know from the beginning of time? No. You just need to learn how to explain the statistics in the project. Linear regression requires knowledge of how to estimate the variability explained by the model (R-squared). As you discuss the results of a Pearson's correlation, one should mention both the test statistic and the p-value associated with it. Translating the symbols in the statistical output into the English language, makes it to easier discuss.

## LEARN THE SYMBOLS

You should know symbols that are part of the writeup. It is not necessary to memorize how-to calculations, but the interpretation should be second nature. Table 7.1 describes the parameters one should be familiar with when analyzing the data. Some symbols are typically reported while others are part of the territory. It is good to be able to explain symbols in your own language. Saying things aloud and learning the language will help your mind accept that you must speak it.

**TABLE 7.1 STATISTICAL SYMBOLS, STATISTICAL METHODS, AND MEANINGS**

| SYMBOL | STATISTICAL METHOD | MEANING |
|---|---|---|
| ρ , r | Pearson's correlations | The magnitude and direction of the relationship between two variables. The range is between -1 to 1. Know which values suggest a negative or positive relationship. Also recognize the strength of the relationship. |
| t | t-distribution | The test statistics used when the standard deviation is unknown, or the sample size is smaller than 30. |
| Df | Degrees of Freedom | The number of values that are free to vary around the sample mean. |
| α | Alpha | Rejection criteria for a hypothesis test |
| F | F statistic | Test statistic used for an ANOVA. |
| β | Linear regression and Type II error | Parameters estimate to describe the behavior of an independent variable versus the outcome measure. Also, the reference is used for other statistical calculations such as power calculations. |
| $X^2$ | Chi square test | Test statistics for data which are illustrated in a contingency table. |
| N | Sample size | Sample Size |
| $\bar{x}$ | Sample mean | Sample mean |

Some of the symbols are used interchangeably among several test statistics. The Cronbach's alpha and the criteria for rejecting the null, refer to an *alpha.* It is helpful to frame your interpretation with a point of reference. The beta symbol for a linear regression parameter is not the same statistic as the type II error for a power of the test. Your best bet is to question every symbol in the output. A notebook of decodes may help one remember certain phrases and definitions. Have fun with it! Knowing the translation, will make it easy to speak the language with confidence.

**EXPLAIN IT TO SOMEONE ELSE**

Knowledge of a subject is half the battle; one should be able to articulate what they understand. Speaking it aloud to someone forces one to run through the logic in the interpretation. The author learned a lot of complex statistical methods through teaching others, especially if the audience gives feedback on the explanation. The more you practice explaining the different symbols and calculations, the easier it will be to present them to an audience. Statistics is not something that you can memorize. If you are familiar with the concepts, it is easier to talk organically about it. Table 7.1 goes over suggested exercises to help one become comfortable with speaking the language of statistics.

TABLE 7.1 EXERCISES FOR SPEAKING THE LANGUAGES OF STATISTICS

| Topic | Exercises | How it Helps |
|---|---|---|
| Linear Regression | Explain which variables are statistically significant to the model. Interpret the R square. Explain how to interpret the Beta Estimates of each variable. | Clears any confusion about which variables are significant to the dependent variable. |
| Chi-Square Test | Interpret the p-value. Explain what the results suggest in terms of associations of the variables. Is there an association? | Helps you remember what details are important for the statistical method. |
| Cronbach's Alpha | Interpret the alpha statistic. What does it suggest in terms of the items in the survey tool? What is considered a satisfactory value for the test statistic? | Helps you discuss whether the items of the survey agree. |

**REFLECTIVE QUESTIONS**

1. Rate the explanation on a scale of 1 to 3 (1=Makes no sense; 2=I am not sure; 3=Makes Sense).

   a. The sample was represented by 120% of the patients.

   b. Of the population, 0.13 are smokers.

   c. The mean difference in body temperature is 50%.

   d. The results are not statistically significant with a p-value of 0.789.

   e. There are 40% Caucasians, 60% Asian and Pacific Islander, and 90% Other in the sample.

2. Do you know the meaning behind your statistical output?
3. What probability distribution chart is used for a Student-t-test?
4. What probability distribution chart is used for an ANOVA?
5. Can you name the test statistic used to perform your analysis in the project?
6. What is the sampling method used for data collection in the project?
7. What is the sample size and how many different characteristics were collected in the spreadsheet?
8. What is your outcome measure and variable type?

# CHAPTER 8

# HOLDING COURT: PRESENT YOUR DATA

In previous chapters we established that it is the DNP researcher's responsibility to know the statistical output. Getting comfortable with the material will help prepare for a Microsoft PowerPoint presentation of the project. The PowerPoint slides serve as the key highlights of the project. Sometimes people use the slides as an outline to stay on topic. Other people feel comfortable talking without looking at the slides. If you are nervous about the presentation, be sure you are familiar with the slides.

## YOU KNOW IT . . . BECAUSE YOU DID IT

The one thing to remember is that the DNP researcher knows the most about his or her project. It helps to think about all the late nights spent writing the manuscript, or the challenges faced with recruiting the participants. The intervention implemented was the DNP researcher's decision and, in some cases, their brainchild. So, there is no reason to doubt your knowledge of the project. Presentation is an opportunity to share your experience with an audience. Before the presentation, any deviations from the original proposal were explained. Any issue with the data was handled and resolved. All missing data is accounted for in the slide presentation. You are simply recounting the experience with the project and summarizing any discussion points.

## HOW TO SAY, "I DON'T KNOW," WITHOUT SEEMING CLUELESS.

There will always be a situation where an audience member poses a question that catches one off guard. The best approach is to remain transparent. If the question is out of your scope, admit to it. There is nothing wrong with recommending more research is needed to answer that question. Any limitations to the project could be highlighted in the presentation. Doing so shows an ability to think critically about the problem areas that need improvement.

### STICK TO THE SLIDES

The slide presentation should contain the sample size, the summary statistics, graphs, and featured statistical method results. You can take the information directly from your manuscript. Any limitations to the project should go in the presentation. The objective of the slides is to provide a briefing of the project details. The graphs are more readable as screen shots than copy and paste. Figure 8.1 is an example of an unreadable graph. The PowerPoint slide should be large enough to see the details of x and y axis.

**FIGURE 8.1 AN UNREADABLE GRAPH**

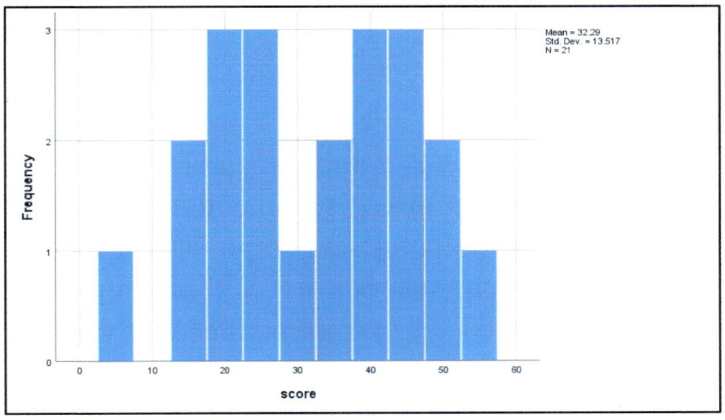

FIGURE 8.2 DISORGANIZED PRESENTATION SLIDE

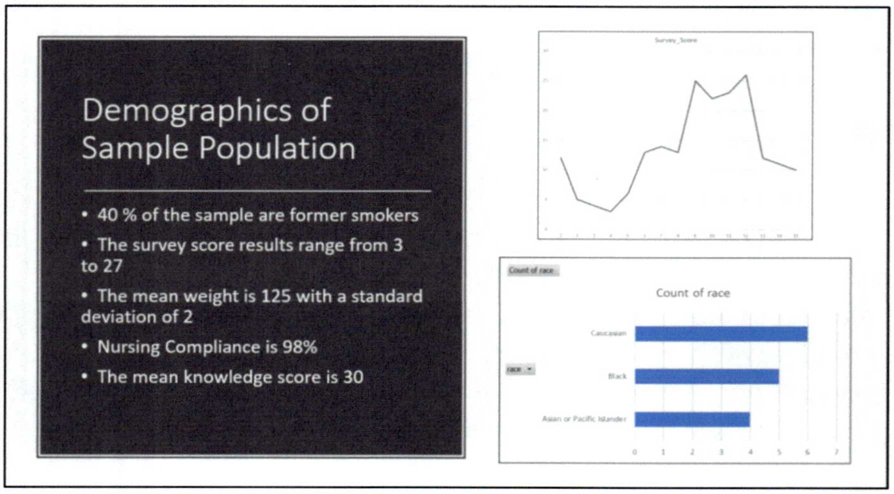


Another typical mistake is to put too many themes on the same slide. Figure 8.2 shows an example of a slide that contains commentary for data that is not in the graphs. The commentary in the slides should speak about the illustrations. If you mention the compliance rate, it might be advantageous to display a weekly compliance rate graph. It is great that Microsoft PowerPoint has so many choices, but it must make sense. Well organized slides result in fewer questions. Before everything is finalized, it is recommended that you practice the presentation in slide mode. It is important to critique the presentation from the perspective of the audience.

### AN OFFENSE IS BETTER THAN NO DEFENSE

After the slides are finalized, try to identify weak areas. At the presentation stage, you know the limitations of the project. It is better to present the project with transparency and discuss the missing data or non-compliancy issues. The data will tell a story whether it is addressed or not. Metaphorically speaking, it's like the data is the side kick who will either support your narrative or contradict it. If the findings are not statistically significant, corresponding tables or figures should be omitted from the presentation. By presenting weak data, you are requiring the audience to digest an unimportant visual.

### LAST COMMENTARY ON SLIDES

It has already been established that one should only provide graphs which have significant findings. It has been the author's experience that approximately twenty-five slides should equal an hour-long presentation. Of course, timing depends on the number of questions from the audience. It might be valuable to make recommendations for future projects with similar themes. Remember that any project limitations can be corrected in future published works.

**REFLECTIVE QUESTIONS**

1. How many themes are mentioned on each slide?
2. Did you cover the limitations of your project in terms of the data?
3. Ask a peer to look at your slides. Is each slide self-explanatory?
4. Are there slides which do not answer the research question?
5. Do you know all the statistical symbols on the slides?

# CHAPTER 9

# TALKING TO THE ROYAL COURT

This chapter is a compilation of the many experiences one has witnessed with the DNP projects and the PhD dissertation process. At some point, it is important to check in with faculty concerning your progress with the data. Some nursing schools will divide the classes by milestones. There may be an IRB course to assess the scientific nature of the work. There may be a literature review course that addresses issues with that component of the manuscript. Other nursing programs require the student to work more independently. In every scenario, the nursing student must organize and execute the task. Some faculty will assist you with the organization of the project. She or he may spend countless hours editing the wording of a phrase or critiquing the detail of the analysis. Other programs may not have specialized support for their students.

## FACULTY AND PEERS

Conversations with faculty and peers have an influence on the fate of your project. Faculty will provide insight regarding weaknesses in the execution of the work. If the sample size calculation is vague or missing, a professor will tell you. Perhaps there is a situation where the details of the proposal need to be pivoted due to the coronavirus. Discussions with faculty immediately impact the project. Peer review of the project can be helpful and harmful at the same time. You do not need to add a graph or test statistic to compete with other students. There may be a reason why your colleague did not need an inference test for their write up. However, it is helpful to get honest feedback from a friend who can relate to the struggle of the process.

## HOW TO PREPARE FOR A DISCUSSION ABOUT YOUR DATA

Meetings with faculty are of the utmost importance. If the conversation is about data collection tools, the Excel spreadsheet should be ready for presentation. Be prepared to answer questions about the data. How will you collect the dairy cards? Have you worked out the logistics of monitoring the nursing compliance on a weekly basis? Is it feasible to do a retrospective chart review on 1000 patients in two weeks? Is the research topic doable given the current state of healthcare? Table 9.1 shows a data analysis cheat sheet for your upcoming meeting. The task list will depend upon the phase of the project and the facility.

TABLE 9.1 DATA PREPARATION FOR FACULTY MEETING

| TASK | PHASE OF STUDY | DETAIL TO KNOW |
|---|---|---|
| Excel Spreadsheet Design | Proposal Stage | - Variable names and formats<br>- Data Storage<br>- De-identification process |
| Sample Size and Sampling Size | Proposal Stage | - Statistical method used for analysis<br>- Sampling method<br>- Outcome measure<br>- Independent variables |
| Graphs and Tables of Data | Manuscript | - Clearly defined x and y axis<br>- P-values clearly labeled<br>- Ensure the data answers the research question. |
| Validation of Survey/Implementation Tool | Proposal | - Cronbach's Alpha from literature if applicable<br>- Calculation of survey tool<br>-Number of constructs under study |

Preparation for meeting calls are fundamental. If the objective of the meeting is to discuss inclusion criteria, one would prepare to discuss the age range and other details of the participants. It is unwise to come to a meeting with an implementation tool and no validation statistics. If the survey tool has been utilized by others in the past, more than likely there is a Cronbach's alpha associated with the survey tool. Some *instruments* come with algorithms for scoring participants. It is the author's opinion that the meeting will go smoother if a pre-existing tool is chosen for the project. New implementation tools require a series of validation steps that are out of the scope of this book. Reliability analysis of Cronbach's alpha is only one aspect of survey tool validation.

**FUTURE WORKS: PUBLICATIONS**

It is good to plan for future analysis. What would you do differently? Are there limitations in the project that could be explored on a deeper level? Some nursing projects are conducted in an environment that is not conducive for data collection. The author's advice is to brainstorm about the issues that one faces during this pandemic. New restrictions have arisen from the coronavirus. Data queens everywhere are noting the limitations of conducting their projects remotely. The hope is that we will devise new methods for addressing the need of medical staff, patient, and healthcare. Get excited about data!

### Reflective Questions

1. Are you prepared for your meeting with faculty?
2. Can you articulate the weaknesses of the project?
3. Do you know how the data will be collected, analyzed, and reported?
4. If this meeting is about the research topic, do you have alternative topics?
5. Do you feel like a Data Queen now?

# Glossary

| | |
|---|---|
| Chi-Square Distribution | A distribution specifically used for count data |
| confidence interval | Is the range of possible values given the point estimate and level of confidence |
| convenience sampling | Sampling based on data which is easily obtainable, such as, a doctor's office |
| data | The source of organized information in the form of variables (columns) and observations (rows) is data |
| dependent variable | The variable which is predicted by the independent variable. |
| DNP | Doctorate of Nursing Practice |
| frequency | Counting the number of times, a value appears in the data |
| independent variable | The variable which is free to vary within your statistical model. |
| IRB | Stands for Institutional Review Board which monitors biomedical research under the Federal Drug Administration guidelines |
| low limit | Is value which represents the minimum value of your threshold |
| mean | A calculation which represents the typical value of in data |

| | |
|---|---|
| Measures of central tendency | Statistics that summarize what is a typical value that represents your data |
| median | Value which represents the 50% mark where half the ordered data is below and above it. |
| mode | Most frequent value in your data. |
| Normal Distribution | The distribution for interval or ratio data |
| probability sampling | The use of likelihood to determine the members of the population |
| p-value | The probability value that determines statistical significance of a test. |
| R | A Statistical Software Package |
| random sampling | Sampling where each member has an equal likelihood of being chosen for the data collection. |
| range | The distance between your minimum and maximum values |
| sample population | The act of collecting a subset of data from a larger population. |
| SAS | Statistical Analysis Software |
| STATA | Statistics and Data Software |
| STATCrunch | A Statistical Software Package |
| standard deviation | Average distance from the mean or the squared root of the variance |
| true population | The group that contains all the possible members of the population. |
| upper limit | Is value which represents the maximum value of your threshold |
| values | The answers collected for each variable question in your data |

| | |
|---|---|
| variable | The entity which can describe numbers, characters, or symbols. |
| variable format | The uniform appearance of your variables |
| variable type | The variable characteristic which determines its analysis: ordinal, nominal, ratio, or interval |
| variance | The noise in your data. The spread from the mean. |

Made in the USA
Monee, IL
03 May 2026

49396328R00033